Dear Stacia,

You have a beautiful spirit — and an awesome smile! Continue to enjoy your life!

With Style & Amazing Grace

May the Lord continue to bless you!

Warmly,
Aleysha Proctor

With Style & Amazing Grace

Style & Beauty Really Does Start on the Inside and Is Seen On the Outside

∞

ALEYSHA R. PROCTOR

Copyright © 2007 by Aleysha R. Proctor.

Library of Congress Control Number:		2007902594
ISBN:	Hardcover	978-1-4257-6384-8
	Softcover	978-1-4257-6366-4

All rights reserved. No part of this book may be reproduced or transmitted in any form or by any means, electronic or mechanical, including photocopying, recording, or by any information storage and retrieval system, without permission in writing from the copyright owner.

This book was printed in the United States of America.

To order additional copies of this book, contact:
Xlibris Corporation
1-888-795-4274
www.Xlibris.com
Orders@Xlibris.com

Contents

Introduction   7
With Gratitude   11
What Is Style?   15
What Is Grace?   25
How to BE   33
What Are You Thinking About?   41
The Spirit of Excellence   49
The Beauty of Creating   59
A Leader Worth Following   69
The Simple Life   77
Your Best Accessory   85
Strength While You're Waiting   91
Oh—To Be Thankful!   99
The Wellness Factor   107
. . . and Amen   115

Introduction

It is with great pleasure that I pen down my first book. For years, people have asked me when I was going to write a book, at first, I didn't think that I had much to say. However, over the last few years, the Lord has really been working in my life, and I knew that I needed to share some of the things that He's worked out inside of me.

It's my prayer that this book will help someone live a more fulfilling life, and to not get discouraged along the journey—there's hope!

Romans 15:13 tells us, "Now may the God of **hope** fill you with all joy and peace in believing, that you may abound in **hope** by the power of the Holy Spirit."

In "With Style & Amazing Grace" we start on the outward appearance, go inside and then come back out. In Chapter 1 we talk about personal style and what colors may be best for you—but we can't dress up a disaster that's brewing on the inside of us. So, we deal with that too!

In Chapter 2, we talk about what Grace is and how to be Graceful.

In Chapter 3, we discuss how to really be a Human Being. In Chapter 4, I'd like to challenge your thinking, and help you to create a better world around you.

In Chapter 5, we discuss the Spirit of Excellence, what it is and what it isn't and who can have it! Hmmm . . . good stuff!

We then go on to discuss how we can create the life of our dreams—making your dreams your reality. And then there's the subject of leadership—you'll want to read this closely. Leadership may not be what you think it is!

"And, oh, The Simple Life, we talk about making good decisions."

And how about a person's Best Accessory? Hmmm . . . I wonder what that could be!

In the next chapter, you'll learn how to bask in the beauty of waiting! Yes, WAITING!

Next, we show you how to go "over the top" in life! Who doesn't want to do that?! We then discuss taking care of your physical temple.

And lastly, it's Amen and so be it!

By applying the principles in this book, you should find solutions to the six major aspects of your life: spiritual, mental, physical, emotional, financial and relational.

With Gratitude

Of course, my first Special Thanks goes to my Lord and Savior Jesus Christ, from Whom all blessings flow!

Next, I'd like to say thank you to my mother, Merriell E. Briscoe who has been an example of strength for me throughout my entire life. To my sister, best friend and business partner, Anjela E. Proctor who has always been a sounding board and a constant advisor to me (you need people like this in your life!)

To my brother, Derek, who keeps me on my toes! To my stepdad, Eddie for always being there. To Grandmother Scott who always has a word of encouragement.

To my aunts & uncles and other family members who always seem to think that I'll do the right thing. Thank you!

To my God-Sister, Tonya Y. Lewis, who always believes that I can do anything. Thank you!

To my Warm Spirit business team—*The Blue Chip Society Team*—who keeps me humble and grateful to the Lord for His blessings!

To my church family at the First Baptist Church of Glenarden Maryland—a ministry of Excellence.

And to you, for reading this book,
THANK YOU!

What Is Style?

What is Style? I'm so glad that you asked! I could go through a long definition of what the word "style" means, but the short answer is style is BEING YOURSELF ON PURPOSE!

Your style is your own signature. It's unique, it's why you do what you do. It's your personal style and lifestyle rolled into one.

Understanding your own personal style takes time to know what you REALLY like and what works well for you. What works well for the image that you're trying to get across to others, not the image that you're trying to fit into for, maybe, a job or a position. But at the end of the day, who are you?

Have you ever been out shopping and you see a handbag or a jacket or a shade of lipstick and you say, "Aunt Susie would like that. That looks like something that she would wear?" That's because you recognize Aunt Susie's personal style. Whether you agree with it or not, it's hers.

Style should not be confused with fashion. Style says, "I need to be comfortable, and what works for me in this particular occasion." Fashion says, "I know those shoes will kill my feet, but they're the latest thing right now" or "Since they make this dress in my size, then I should wear it."

So how does one discover their own personal style? It takes time. It takes a conscious effort. Take time and notice what others around you are wearing. Is this something that would work well for you too? What comes to mind when you think of Hollywood legends like Audrey Hepburn or Grace Kelly? Those women had great personal style and they knew what worked for them.

Today, we could look at Jada Pinkett Smith, Nicole Kidman and Halle Berry. Whether they're dressed for the red carpet or out in sports wear—they always look great. Why? Because they know what works well for them and their body shapes. They look pulled together, not thrown together.

Looking great in your own style isn't really determined by your budget. You can look stylish in items that were given to you or things that you've purchased from your favorite stores, whether they're expensive department stores or inexpensive catalogs.

Generally, Style falls into four different categories:

Natural
Romantic
Classic
Dramatic

And, I'd like to propose yet, another, Style category and that's Casual Elegance.

How do you know which one you fit into? Take a look at the description categories on the next page and determine which one best describes you. Everyone may find themselves in ALL of the categories, but there's ONE that's your dominant style.

PERSONAL STYLE

Which One Are You?

A. Casual, Relaxed, Confident, Hair is low-maintenance; likes clothing to be casually tailored.

B. Softly Sophisticated, Receptive, Charming, Approachable; likes clothing to be flowing or fitted.

C. Controlled, Poised, Polished, Always Appropriate; likes clothing to be tailored.

D. Sophisticated, Formal, Makes a Statement; likes clothing to be bold and high-fashion.

E. Relaxed, Graceful, Always Appropriate, Confident; likes clothing to be comfortable and stylish.

If you answered Category:

- A. Natural
- B. Romantic
- C. Classic
- D. Dramatic
- E. Casual Elegance

NATURALS: Aren't fussy over their hair and make-up. Their hair may be naturally textured and/or colored. Their clothing is comfortable and casual.

ROMANTICS: Are fussy over hair and make-up. They like to wear clothing with ruffles and floral prints, may be flowing or fitted. After all, they're thinking about Romance!

CLASSICS: Are always polished, tailored and professional looking. Their hair and make-up is usually flawless.

DRAMATICS: Like to wear bold clothes that make a statement. Their hair and make-up usually makes a statement too.

CASUAL ELEGANCE: Are somewhat of a mix between Naturals & Classics. They're always appropriate, but more relaxed that Classics. Hair and make-up is usually flawless.

The Importance of Color

Just a quick word about color. It's important that you know and wear the colors that are right for you. Colors have a way of making you look and feel better, but the wrong colors can make you feel depressed and not look your best.

When someone gets his or her "colors done", they normally fit into one of four seasonal categories: Spring, Summer, Autumn or Winter.

You can do your own self color analysis, but it's best if done by a color or image consultant.

Look at the color of your hair, eyes and skin. The combination of the three will be either Warm or Cool.

Warm

Hair: Blond, Auburn, Brown, Light Brown, Red

Eyes: Warm Brown, Hazel, Light Brown, shades of Green

Skin: Look for the undertones, are they warm (golden or yellow)?

Cool

Hair: Black, Grey, White, Silver

Eyes: Black, Dark Brown, shades of Blue.

Skin: Again, look at the undertones. Do you see blue, pink or red?

People who are considered "Springs" or "Autumns" are Warm, and those who are "Summers" and "Winters" are Cool.

Warm Colors of Choice: Gold, Browns, Ivories, Greens, shades of Orange, shades of Yellow.

Cool Colors of Choice: Silver, Black, Whites, Reds, Blues, Fuchsia, shades of Purple.

Neutrals: Some people also fall into a "neutral" palette. Those with a combination of cool and warm color, such as me. While my hair and eyes are definitely cool, my skin tone is warm.

For all of the Neutrals out there—what colors do you think work best for you? You've got it! Neutrals! Such as Silver, Gold, Camel, Taupe, Black, Navy and Beige. Coral and Turquoise are universal colors and can be worn by all color palettes.

So, now you're aware of your style and what colors may be best for you. Now, let's talk about what's going on inside of you.

Aleysha Recommends

Since I am also a certified image consultant, I can't talk about style and not say something about your wardrobe.

Suggested Wardrobe Basics:

White Button-Up Shirt
White T-shirt or Shell
Denim Jacket
Black Skirt
Black Pants
Pair of Jeans
Scarf or Wrap
Black Dress (for all occasions)
Colorful Blouse
Cardigan twin-set or Jacket

With these recommended pieces, comes a whole wardrobe:

White Button-Up Blouse with Black Pants
White Button-Up Blouse with Black Skirt
White Button-Up Blouse with Jeans
Colorful Blouse with Black Pants
Colorful Blouse with Black Skirt
Twinset with Black Pants
Twinset with Black Skirt
Twinset with Jeans
Black Dress with Cardigan (from twinset)
Denim Jacket, White t-shirt, Black Pants
Denim Jacket, White t-shirt, Black Skirt

You get the idea!
You can have an entire wardrobe just by mixing and matching these ten items.

In What Areas Would You Like to Improve?

What Is Grace?

Ahhhh . . . . Grace.

"But He gives more grace. Wherefore He said, "God resists the proud, but gives grace to the humble". James 4:6

First of all, Grace from God is a gift! It's favor—it's provisions to do things beyond your own abilities. We should all want more grace in our lives!

But what does it mean to be Graceful? I once had a gentleman friend who told me that I was graceful—at that time, I didn't quite know what he meant, but I knew that it was a great compliment. So, of course, I wanted to know more about grace and being graceful. Here's what I found out.

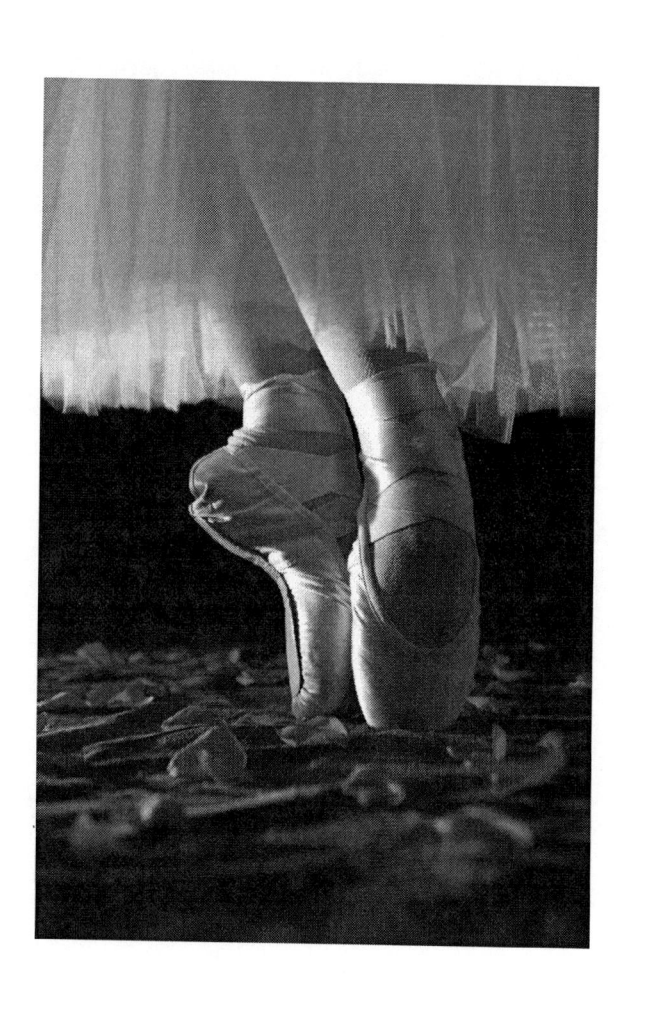

Graceful means to show beauty in form and/or movement, to be elegant, to suggest good taste. Think of a ballet dancer or one who plays the violin or piano with such ease.

I was several years younger at the time of this compliment, so I wondered how I became graceful.

In reading James 4:6, my question was answered, "God gives grace to those who are humbled!" I realized that God had made me graceful! I realized that you can speak volumes with a soft voice, and humbly walk into a room and be content to sit in the back and graciously allow someone else to have the spotlight. Grace isn't bestowed on the proud or arrogant, but out of a grateful heart and an obedient spirit comes grace.

Men can also be graceful. The popular actor many years ago, Carey Grant, was once described as a graceful man. He was elegant, charming, seemingly well-mannered and didn't mind making fun of himself and letting someone else appear to be the star. Humble.

The Bible tells us that Noah and Moses found grace in the sight of the Lord. It also says that Jesus was full of grace (graceful) and truth (truthful).

Are you graceful? Do you want to become graceful? If so, then humble yourself and quiet your spirit so that you may hear from the Lord. Realize that all good and perfect gifts come from God—and ask Him to show you how to become more graceful. The grace that the Lord gives starts on the inside of you and is then seen on the outside as being graceful.

Being graceful has its benefits. Have you ever went somewhere, let's say a restaurant and had to wait an extra long time or the kitchen was out of the specials of the day? And maybe the person next to you didn't take the news so well and begins to yell at the waiter for the shortage, or restaurant hostess for the long wait.

Realizing the grace and mercy that God has extended to us should cause us to want to show grace and mercy to someone else.

But being graceful has a quiet and patient demeanor, it's gentle. I've gotten several favors for being patient or understanding in these types of situations, like a better table, better service, a free appetizer or dessert.

You see, in the book of Esther 2:17, it says that Esther found grace AND favor in the sight of the king and he made her queen over Vashti! Being graceful does normally warrant favor!

The squeaky wheel doesn't always get the oil—sometimes silence is golden!

Aleysha Recommends

Read the Book of Esther in the Bible and see what made her graceful and find grace and favor in the sight of the king. What caused her to be crowned queen?

Also, observe someone who you think is graceful and see what they do and how they do it.

In What Areas Would You Like to Improve?

How to BE

Exodus 33: 13-14, "Now therefore, I pray, if I have found grace in Your sight, show me now Your way, that I may know You. And consider that this nation is Your people. And He said, "My Presence will go with you, and I will give you rest."

In this very modern age that we're living in, there's always the thought that you have to be BUSY at all times! I once heard the tele-evangelist Joyce Meyer say that we aren't human doings, we're human beings and need to learn how to just rest and be sometimes.

Even God Himself took time to rest after He created the heavens and the earth and the things in the earth. There are countless scriptures that tell us to rest. In the above passage, God is meeting with Moses. In verse 11a, it says that the Lord spoke with Moses face to face as a man speaks to his friend! Imagine that!! Now, Moses is still in "work mode", asking God to show him His way that he may know Him, but God tells him, that His Presence will go with Moses and He'll give him REST!

Rest is important to the human body because you can only function well when you have energy and you get energized while you're resting. Your spirit also needs time to rest and be renewed.

I'm constantly busy. In any given week, after working all day at my corporate job, I also have a thriving business with several hundred business partners (and growing!), and then I have Board meetings to attend, and receptions to go to and network, I'm active in my church, I receive invitations to grand openings, movie screenings and the like and I plan special events and luncheons on a regular basis. Oh yes, I'm quite busy! But I also take time to look at my calendar and block days off just to rest and BE! I can't be of much service to God and others when I'm tired, overwhelmed and frazzled—and neither can you. So do yourself and others a favor and learn how to BE and just rest sometimes. All of the busyness will be there when you're rejuvenated again.

Time to Rest

A friend once sent me an email that elaborated on Psalms 23. We've all heard it a million times and have probably quoted it just as much.

But, since we're talking about rest, read this and then close your eyes and meditate on the Lord and all of His provision towards us.

Psalms 23

"The Lord is my shepherd."—That's Relationship!

"I shall not want."—That's Supply!

"He makes me to lie down in green pastures."—That's Rest!

"He leads me besides the still waters."—That's Refreshment!

"He restores my soul."—That's Healing!

"He leads me in the paths of righteousness."—That's Guidance!

"For His name's sake."—That's Purpose!

"Yes, though I walk through the valley of the shadow of death."—That's Testing!

"I will fear no evil."—That's Protection!

"For You are with me."—That's Faithfulness!

"Your rod and Your staff, they comfort me."—That's Comfort!

"You prepare a table before me in the presence of my enemies."—That's Hope!

"My cup runs over."—That's Abundance!

"Surely, goodness and mercy shall follow me all the days of my life."—That's Blessings!

"And I will dwell in the house of the Lord."—That's Security!

"Forever."—That's Eternity!

What else could we possibly need?!

Aleysha Recommends

Do you need to chill out?

Set aside some time to just rest for a while—and don't feel guilty while doing so.

Create your own serenity spa in your home with some Warm Spirit® products. Take a bath in Warm Spirit's Lavender Bath Crystals, with a soy candle lit. Next, place an herbal spa wrap in the microwave for 60 seconds, then place around your shoulders while you have some Easy Time tea (and the candle is still burning) and journal—write down your thoughts and ideas or just sit in quietness. For more information about Warm Spirit® products, visit *www.warmspirit.org/aleysha*.

In What Areas Would You Like to Improve?

What Are You Thinking About?

Philippians 4:8, "Finally, brothers (and sisters), whatever things are true, whatever things are noble, whatever things are just, whatever things are pure, whatever things are lovely, whatever things are of good report, if there is any virtue and if there is anything praiseworthy—think on these things."

What are you thinking about? The Bible has many scriptures that challenge us in our areas of thinking.

Proverbs 27:3 says that whatever you're thinking in your heart—that's what you are! Wow! Why is this important? Because you REALLY do have the ability to shape your life with the things that you desire, but it starts in your thinking.

What we think about, we bring about. Thoughts become things.

As the scriptures above tells us, Philippians 4:8, we should be spending our time thinking about things that are WORTHWHILE! Look at it, whatever is TRUE, NOBLE, JUST, PURE, LOVELY, OF GOOD REPORT, IS THERE ANY VIRTUE, IS IT WORTHY OF PRAISE? If so, then these are the things that you should be thinking about.

The Bible goes on to tell us that out of the abundance of the heart, the mouth will speak (Matthew 12:34b). Remember, earlier we said that what you're thinking in your heart is what you are, and now the Bible is telling us that we'll start to speak out of our mouths INTO THE UNIVERSE what's in our hearts.

Let's look at it again, out of the ABUNDANCE of the heart (whether good or bad)—the mouth will speak. How did the thoughts in your heart become abundant?

You've thought about it A LOT (whatever you think in your heart . . .) Whatever thoughts you've focused on are now in your heart—in abundance—and any day now, you're going to start talking about it. (You're going to start speaking your thoughts—watch out now!) Mark 11:23 tells us that we shall have what we say.

Luke 6:45 says, "A good man out of the good treasure of his **heart** brings forth that which is good; and an evil man out of the evil treasure of his **heart** brings forth that which is evil: for out of the **abundance of the heart** his mouth speaks."

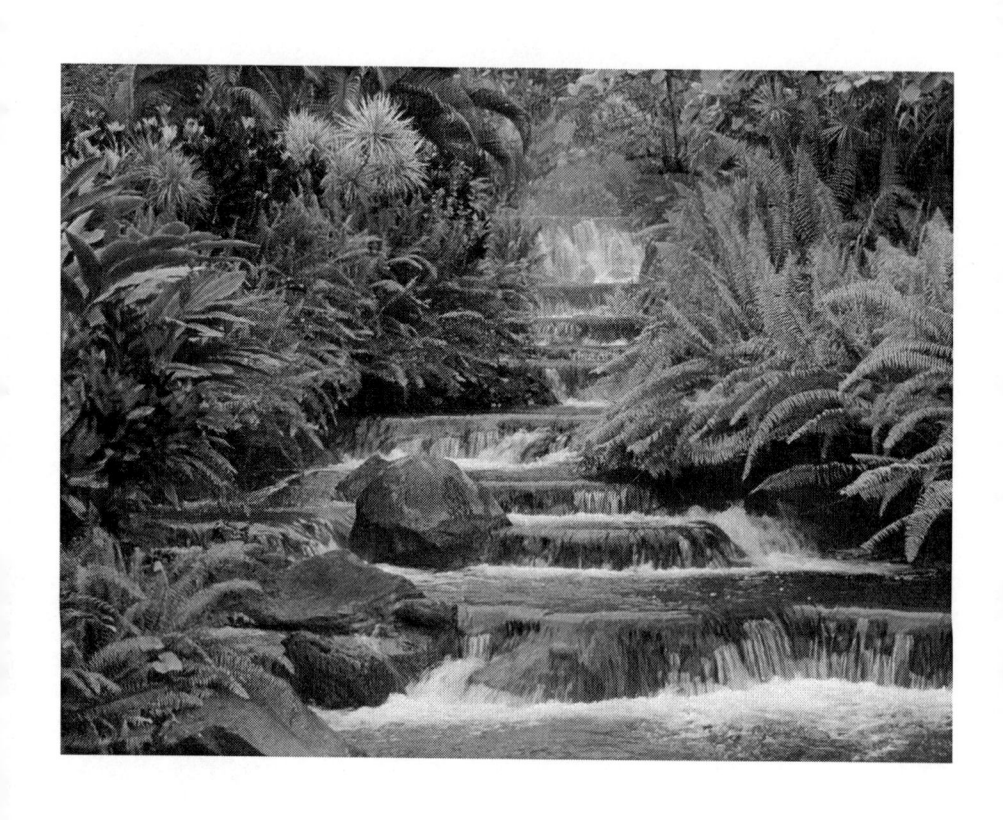

So, if your thinking isn't right or of a good report, you'll want to change it quickly because you'll start to talk about what you're thinking and your words and thoughts will begin to shape your life and the things around you!

How do you change your thinking? It first starts with a DECISION to change your thinking. You may need to stop watching television, stop reading the gossip section, stop reading the newspaper, stop reading lustful or violent novels, stop talking to those who don't have your best interest in mind and start doing the opposite of what you've been doing.

Whatever is TRUE, whatever is NOBLE, whatever is JUST, whatever is PURE, whatever is LOVELY, whatever is of a GOOD REPORT, if there is any virtue and if there is anything praiseworthy—think on these things!

Aleysha Recommends

Are you having trouble seeing beautiful things in your mind? Try going to an art gallery or a museum and observe the paintings. Maybe you should visit a floral shop and study the flowers, or observe the sky on a bright, sunny day. Maybe you could spend some time sitting in the lobby of the most expensive 5-star hotel in your town and soak up the atmosphere of what makes this hotel grand.

How about going window shopping and browse through the stores that you've always wanted to shop in, but maybe your budget doesn't allow you to purchase from yet.

How about this one: start thinking the best of people.

These things are all free and they can change your thinking if you allow them to.

In What Areas Would You Like to Improve?

The Spirit of Excellence

Proverbs 17:27, "He that has knowledge spares his words; and a man (or woman) of understanding is of an excellent spirit."

Excellence is NOT perfection! Everyone who chooses to be excellent or extraordinary can be—but perfection doesn't exist when we're talking about human beings.

What makes a person excellent or extraordinary? Let's look at the words: excellent—the dictionary defines it as unusual goodness or worth, excelling, an outstanding feature. Extraordinary is just that—putting the 'extras' on what is already the ordinary. Going the extra mile, staying an extra ten minutes at work or spending extra time on a project can make a huge difference.

Excellence doesn't boast—it's humble, but it's seen by all!

Let's look at the book of Daniel for a moment. In Daniel 1:8, it says that Daniel PURPOSED IN HIS HEART that he wouldn't defile himself. In other words, he made a DECISION to do what's right and not just to be an ordinary person who's going with the flow.

Let's look further down in Daniel 5, King Belshazzar is having a feast and he and his guests are praising the gods of gold, silver, iron, wood and stone. Out of nowhere, a man's finger appears and begins writing on the wall and King Belshazzar is greatly troubled and afraid. He calls for all of the magicians and soothsayers for them to solve the "handwriting on the wall", but they can't and he's troubled even more.

The queen comes in and tells the king about a man named Daniel, in whom an EXCELLENT spirit is in him. She goes on to say in verse 12, "Inasmuch as an excellent spirit, knowledge, understanding, interpreting dreams, solving riddles, and explaining enigmas were found in THIS Daniel." (Not to be confused with any other Daniels, you understand.)

In verse 13, Daniel is brought before the king. The king spoke and said to Daniel, "Are you THAT Daniel who is one of the captives from Judah, whom my father the king brought from Judah? Verse 14: **I have heard of you**, that the Spirit of God is in you, and that light and understanding and EXCELLENT wisdom are found in you. Verse 15: Now the wise men, the astrologers, have been brought in before me, that they should read this writing and make known to me its interpretation, but they could not give the interpretation of the thing. Verse 16: **And I have heard of you**, that you can give interpretations and explain enigmas. Now, if you can read the writing and make known to me its interpretation, you shall be clothed with a purple robe and have a chain of gold around your neck, and shall be third ruler in the kingdom."

Get the picture! THIS Daniel, who had been taken into captivity, was being bragged on by the queen to the king because it was known that he had an excellent spirit. Now here's this 'prisoner' being brought before the king and the king is offering him gifts and a POSITION IN HIS KINGDOM if he can solve the interpretation. But along with excellence comes humility! And Daniel says in Verse 17: "Let your gifts be for yourself and give your rewards to another; yet I will read the writing to the king and make known to him the interpretation. Verse 18: O king, the Most High God gave Nebuchadnezzar, your father, a kingdom and majesty, glory and honor. Verse 19: And because of the majesty that He gave him, all people, nations, and languages trembled and feared before him. Whomever he wished, he kept alive; whomever he wished, he set up; and whomever he wished, he put down. Verse 20: But when his heart was LIFTED UP, and his spirit was hardened with PRIDE, he was deposed from his kingly throne, and they took his glory from him. Verse 21: Then he was driven from the sons of men, his heart was made like the beasts, and his dwelling was with the wild donkeys. They fed him with grass like oxen, and his body was wet with the dew of heaven, TILL HE KNEW that the Most High God rules in the kingdom of men, and appoints over it whomever He chooses."

Now get this! Verse 22 says, "But you his son, Belshazzar, have NOT HUMBLED YOUR HEART, although you knew all of this. Verse 23: And you have LIFTED YOURSELF UP against the Lord of heaven. They have brought the vessels of His house before you, and you and your lords, your wives and your concubines, have drunk wine from them. And you have praised the gods of silver and gold, bronze, iron, wood and stone; which DO NOT SEE OR HEAR OR KNOW; and (catch this!) the God WHO HOLDS YOUR BREATH IN HIS HAND AND OWNS ALL OF YOUR WAYS, you have not glorified. Verse 24: Then the fingers of the hand were sent from Him (the Lord), and this writing was written. Verse 25: And this is the inscription that was written:

MENE, MENE, TEKEL, PERES.

Verse 26: This is the interpretation of each word. MENE: God has numbered your kingdom, and finished it; Verse 27: TEKEL: you have been weighed in the balances and found wanting; Verse 28: PERES: Your kingdom has been divided, and given to the Medes and Persians. Verse 29: Then Belshazzar gave the command, and they clothed Daniel with purple and put a chain of gold around his neck and made a proclamation concerning that he should be the third ruler in the kingdom."

Look at Verse 6:3 "Then THIS Daniel distinguished himself above the governors and satraps, because an EXCELLENT spirit *was* in him; and the king gave thought to setting him over the whole realm."

Hear me now, let's summarize all of this! Daniel had been taken into captivity (THIS Daniel), but because he PURPOSED in his heart to do what was right and not to defile himself and to obey the Lord (he just made a decision), he had an EXCELLENT spirit in him. The queen is in the palace bragging on Daniel to the king! The king brings Daniel into the palace and says to him TWO TIMES—I have heard of you!

Excellence will cause other people to hear about you and you're not the one doing the bragging!!!

Daniel is humbled by all of the gifts that the king is offering to give him, but asks him to give the gifts to someone else. He goes on to solve the interpretation, which says that, "You have not humbled yourself and you knew what happened to your father and his kingdom when he lifted himself up in pride. So, because you have done the same thing, your kingdom is divided and given to another!

Then in Verse 6:3, Daniel stands out above the other governors and leaders—why? Because an EXCELLENCE spirit is in him—so much so, that the king is thinking of making him #1 in the kingdom!

Isn't that something! Excellence and humility will lift you up, but pride comes before the fall!

People of excellence are praisers—they don't complain and find fault in everything. Remember, earlier we talked about thinking about things that are of a good report and praiseworthy.

People of excellence are purpose-driven. Doing things in an excellent manner is a part of their lifestyle. You don't have to have exceptional talents, intelligence or personality to be a person of excellence. It's a level playing field—anyone can achieve success if they purpose in their hearts to do things in an excellent manner. It's just a matter of choice!

I once heard someone say that when you're mediocre—you're the best of the worst (unsatisfactory to mediocre) and the worst of the best (mediocre to excellent)! Yikes!

In today's terminology, I recall reading the front page of the Washington Post Sports section in late January 2007. The title grabbed my attention, it read, "Butler Chose to be One of the Chosen."

The article went on to say that a Washington Wizard NBA player simply CHOSE to stand out and become an extraordinary athlete. It further went on to say that 'he made it his business to get better at his game during the off season' and work to be chosen to the NBA All-Star game (he went the extra mile!)

He simply made a decision to be a person of excellence.

Choose this day whether you'll be a person of mediocrity or excellence.

Aleysha Recommends

Are you a person of excellence? Would you like to be?

Take inventory of your work ethic. Can you stand to spend extra time at work to put the finishing touches on a project? It was said that Picasso and Michelangelo and other famous painters and sculptors would emphatically put their name onto their artwork, as to say, "THIS IS MY WORK AND I'M PLEASED WITH IT!"

Can you autograph your work with excellence by putting your name and your own personal touches on it? Or do you hope that your boss doesn't know who did the work, so if it's a shoddy job then maybe your colleagues will get blamed for it?

Make a list—what can you do better? What can you give a better effort to? How can you improve on something?

To be a person of excellence, it requires a decision made by you that your work will stand out above others and that you won't be satisfied until you've done your absolute best!

Be determined that you won't be content with the status quo or the ordinary. And then do something about it. Go ahead, be an "extra-miler"!

In What Areas Would You Like to Improve?

The Beauty of Creating

Mark 11:24, "Therefore I say to you, whatever things you **ask** when you pray, **believe** that you **receive** them and you will have them."

The Creative Process: Ask, Believe, Receive.

Isn't it beautiful to know that you can create the life that you want for yourself?!

Many people have heard about the book and DVD entitled, "The Secret". And many people shied away from it saying that it wasn't from God. However, in "The Secret", the authors are speaking about the Law of Attraction—that's the secret!

Let me challenge you here for a moment, who made the Laws of the Universe? God did! Remember, in Genesis when He created the heavens and the earth, and all of the things in the earth? Well, He spoke into existence whatever He wanted to see and when He rested on the seventh day, He had already put everything into place, including the laws that govern the universe.

Laws were put in place by God to create ORDER. Can you imagine what your life would be like if there weren't such laws that said that if someone breaks into your home, they stand the chance of going to jail because they've broken the law? If there were no boundaries, no law and order, then we'd have total chaos!

Do you believe in the Law of Gravity? What goes up, must come down.

How about the Law of Giving & Receiving (or the Law of Reciprocity)? Jesus said, "Give and it shall be given back to you."

How about the Law of Cause & Effect? If you eat donuts every day, expect to put on extra weight.

So, why not embrace the Law of Attraction as something from the Lord as well?

Look at the promise that God made to Abraham—which is still in effect today!

Genesis 26: 4, "And I will make your descendants multiply as the stars of heaven; I will give to your descendants all these lands; and in your seed all the nations of the earth shall be blessed; Verse 5 because Abraham obeyed My voice and kept My charge, My commandments, My statutes, and My laws."

God made this "blockbuster" promise to Abraham because what? He obeyed the voice of the Lord and kept His charge, commandments, statues and LAWS.

In "The Secret", the authors say that the Law of Attraction is summed up in three words, Ask—Believe—Receive. In Mark 11:24, Jesus Himself says this!

And again, the scriptures tell us that whatever we think in our hearts, that's what we are. So, if you don't like what you have, then change your thinking! Abundant living starts in your thinking, and so do the things that you're attracting (or drawing) to yourself—whether good or bad.

In the Book of Job, there is a powerful example of the Law of Attraction. It's quite devastating how it worked out in Job's case.

In the very first chapter of Job, servant after servant came to Job with very bad news, as a matter of fact, before the first servant could finish delivering the bad news, here comes another servant with bad news, and before that person could finish speaking, here comes another servant with bad news. Wow! Who could handle such a mountain of bad news at one time like that?! Let's look at it:

Job 1:13, "Now there was a day when Job's sons and daughters *were* eating and drinking wine in their oldest brother's house; **14** and a messenger came to Job and said, "The oxen were plowing and the donkeys feeding beside them, **15** when the Sabeans raided *them* and took them away—indeed they have killed the servants with the edge of the sword; and I alone have escaped to tell you!" **16** While he *was* still speaking, another also came and said, "The fire of God fell from heaven and burned up the sheep and the servants, and consumed them; and I alone have escaped to tell you!" **17** While he *was* still speaking, another also came and said, "The Chaldeans formed three bands, raided the camels and took them away, yes, and killed the servants with the edge of the sword; and I alone have escaped to tell you!" **18** While he *was* still speaking, another also came and said, "Your sons and daughters *were* eating and drinking wine in their oldest brother's house, **19** and suddenly a great wind came from across the wilderness and struck the four corners of the house, and it fell on the young people, and they are dead; and I alone have escaped to tell you!"

How devastating!

Job is then stricken with painful boils from his head to the soles of his feet. He goes out to mourn and his three friends come to mourn with him. In Chapter 3, Job curses the day that he was born and he says something that's very interesting. In verse 25 he says, "For the thing I greatly feared has come upon me, And what I dreaded has happened to me."

Fear starts in your thinking. You begin to think about unfortunate things that may happen to you, and then you begin to fear those things. And just like with positive thinking, you'll also attract the things that you fear to you.

You really do have the power to create—God gave that power to you!

Imagine that!

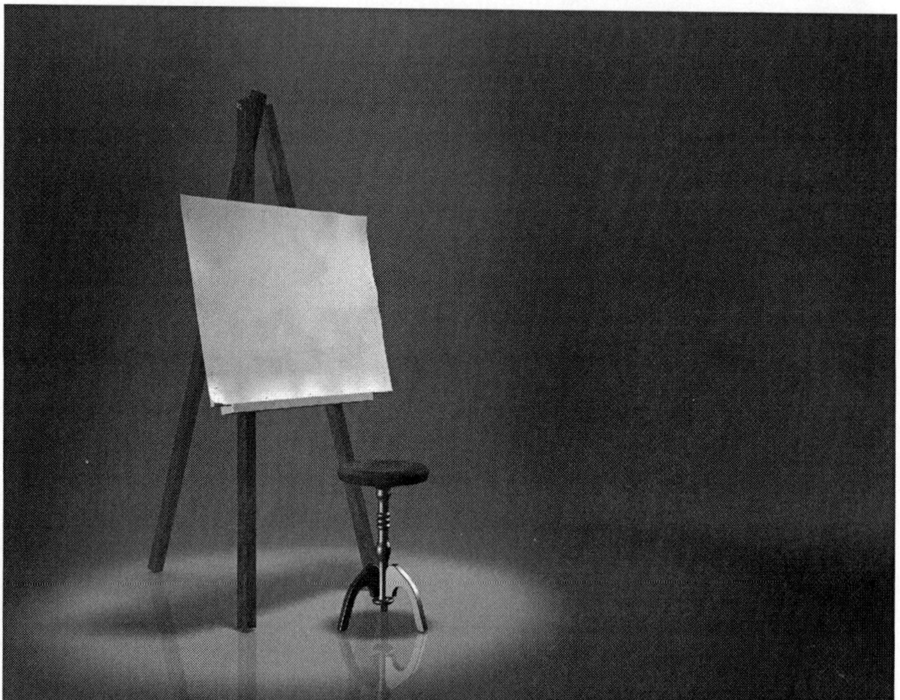

Aleysha Recommends

Take an inventory of your life, do you like what you see? If not, then find an area that you'd like to see changes in. Begin thinking about what those changes would look like in your mind, then start to talk about it (you may have to talk to yourself). Then write down the end result and what your life will look like when the changes occur. Now figure out what you need to do to get you from here to there.

For example, do you like the way that your financial situation looks? Okay, see what having an abundance looks like in your mind, does it mean that you're happier when the bills come in because you know that you have the resources to pay or eliminate them? Do you see yourself driving a better car, living in a better neighborhood, being able to help others out who are in need, eating at the finest restaurants in town, travelling?

You may need a visual to help you with your thinking. How about making a dream board or a dream photo album by cutting out pictures of things you'd like to draw into your life? Make a copy of a check, made payable to you for whatever amount you'd consider to be abundant, find a picture of the car or house that you want and look at it often.

Okay, now, start talking about it. Begin thanking the Lord for your abundant life. Jesus said that He came that we may have life and have it more abundantly!

What does your current bank account look like? Now, what steps will get you from here to there? Maybe it's getting a job that pays more money, or starting a business, or selling things that you have but aren't using.

You don't just have to dream about the things that you want, you can create them for yourself!

In What Areas Would You Like to Improve?

A Leader Worth Following

Matthew 20:25, "But Jesus called them to Himself and said, 'You know that the rulers of the Gentiles lord it over them, and those who are great exercise authority over them. Verse 26: Yet it shall not be so among you; but whoever desires to become great among you, let him be your servant. Verse 27: And whoever desires to be first among you, let him be your slave. Verse 28: Just as the Son of Man did not come to be served, but to serve, and to give His life as a ransom for many."

Leadership is a calling. When you're called to leadership, your life changes because now you have people who depend on you to help make them successful.

People who put themselves into a leadership role may quickly find out that while they may think that they're leading, no one is following them. Why? If those who you're leading feel as though you don't care about them or their success and are only concerned about your own success, they may not follow you.

Leadership calls for you to put yourself on the back-burner and see how you can SERVE those that you're leading.

Doesn't that seem backwards? Shouldn't the followers be serving the leader? According to Christ, whoever wants to be the greatest leader must first learn to become the greatest servant. This is servant-leadership, and it's also leading by example. Your actions are showing your followers how to get the job done.

A leader needs to be mindful of the needs of those who are following them. Why? Because no one can effectively follow someone and carry out the vision and mission that's set forth for the unit, team or organization when they're so weighed down in other matters. Since the leader has oversight of what's going on, he/she needs to see how they can help ease the burdens of their followers so that they can better focus on the mission at hand.

Take for example the leader of a musical band. It's up to the leader to see who needs help in developing their talents so that the band can perform better. Does this mean that you spend extra time with those who need help, or call in additional help to work with those who need it? Whatever it takes to get the job done or the mission accomplished.

Again, this is servant-leadership and leading by example—in this case, the leader is going the extra mile to get the job done.

And leaders, don't worry, you'll get yours! When you help make your followers successful, your success is a done deal!

Don't Forget to Ask For Wisdom

And while you're leading, don't forget to ask for wisdom. Wisdom is an essential part of leadership.

Solomon knew that he'd need wisdom in his new leadership role as king of Israel. In the Bible, God asks him what does he want—can you imagine that—God pretty much giving him a blank check! And Solomon asked for wisdom so that he'd be able to effectively lead the people. God was so impressed with his request that He said, not only will I give you wisdom, but I'm going to give you WHAT YOU DIDN'T ASK FOR— BOTH RICHES AND HONOR!!!

WOW!! So much for God not wanting us to be rich!

Let's look at the text:

I Kings 3:5, "At Gibeon the LORD appeared to Solomon in a dream by night; and God said, "Ask! What shall I give you?" **6** And Solomon said: "You have shown great mercy to Your servant David my father, because he walked before You in truth, in righteousness, and in uprightness of heart with You; You have continued this great kindness for him, and You have given him a son to sit on his throne, as *it is* this day. **7** Now, O LORD my God, You have made Your servant king instead of my father David, but I *am* a little child; I do not know *how* to go out or come in. **8** And Your servant *is* in the midst of Your people whom You have chosen, a great people, too numerous to be numbered or counted. **9** Therefore give to Your servant an understanding heart to judge Your people, that I may discern between good and evil. For who is able to judge this great people of Yours?" **10** The speech pleased the Lord, that Solomon had asked this thing. **11** Then God said to him: "Because you have asked this thing, and have not asked long life for yourself, nor have asked riches for yourself, nor have asked the life of your enemies, but have asked for yourself understanding to discern justice, **12** behold, I have done according to your words; see, I have given you a wise and understanding heart, SO THAT THERE HAS NOT BEEN ANYONE LIKE YOU BEFORE YOU, NOR SHALL ANY LIKE YOU ARISE AFTER YOU. **13 And I have also given you what you have not asked: both riches and honor, so that there shall not be anyone like you among the kings all your days.**

Check that out! God not only fulfilled Solomon's prayer request, and not only did He give him what he didn't ask for (riches and honor)—but God also set Solomon apart from everyone else—God DISTINGUISHED Solomon because He was so impressed with his prayer. God told him, 'So that there has not been anyone like you before you, nor shall any like you arise after you." Whew!!

Look at the text again, Solomon is YOUNG and God ENDOWS him with wisdom (an understanding heart.) This goes to show us that you can be wise at any age, young or old.

You'll need wisdom (an understanding heart) when leading people. Because you need to know how to make long-term decisions and see the "whole" picture, you need to discern what's good and what's not, you'll need to make judgments and decisions that affect other people—and you simply cannot do so effectively without WISDOM.

Do you think that you're lacking in the wisdom department? Again, THERE'S HOPE! All you have to do is ASK for wisdom.

James 1:5 tells us, "If any of you **lacks wisdom**, let him ask of God, who gives to all liberally and without reproach, and it will be given to him."

Aleysha Recommends

Study the life of Christ. He was the ultimate leader—He's still being talked about and impacting lives over 2,000 years later!

What did He do, He came to serve people. His ministry was filled with Him going around healing people (physically, emotionally, mentally, spiritually and financially), He washed the feet of His disciples, He multiplied food so that others could eat, and ultimately, He gave His life so that others may live!

Look at the Book of Esther. See how when she became queen that she put her life on the line so that those in her "queendom" may have their lives spared. She said, "If I perish, then let me perish."

Servant Leadership!

And if you feel that you're lacking in the wisdom department (an understanding heart), which you'll need in your role as a leader, then just ask God for it.

In addition, if you'd like for God to give you a blank check, as He did with Solomon, then pray sincere prayers from your heart that will get His attention and impress Him!

In What Areas Would You Like to Improve?

The Simple Life

I find my time to be very important, and I'm sure that you feel the same way about your time. Therefore, I have to be cognizant as to how I'm spending it. You know the saying, "Time is Money?" Well, it's true. So, if you're wasting your time are you also wasting your money?

I love to live a simple life. You see, to be complicated and complex takes a lot of time and energy, and I only have 24 hours per day. So, I need to get a lot done in a relatively short period of time—plain and simple.

Living a simple life is far from being simple-minded—far, far from it. It just means that you can get more done and you can enjoy your life and the time that you have. Let me give you an example, I have long, thick hair (for which, I'm very grateful to the Lord for!) And I don't have a lot of time for complicated, high-maintenance hairstyles. I have a standing appointment every two weeks with my beautician and whatever hairstyle that I choose to get, I need to be able to maintain it—simply—until my next visit. It would take too much time adding products and having to curl my hair each day, even putting rollers in my hair at night is time consuming—so I need to go to sleep, get up and comb it and be on my way. But it has to be beautiful, you understand.

Another example is my make-up. I mainly choose neutral colors so that I don't have to wipe off one color and reapply make-up should I need to change my clothes throughout the day—it needs to be simple, I don't want to have to pour a lot of time, energy and thought into it, but again, it has to be beautiful and tastefully done.

As women, we tend to be more high-maintenance and complex than men, and sometimes we wonder why they seem to get more accomplished, say, in business, than we do. It's because they don't waste a lot of time in their thought processes. They, usually, can make a decision and stick with it. They can find a system that works well for them and so be it! We, women, tend to overcomplicate matters with being indecisive and wanting to reinvent the wheel for the sake of being creative, which could be a waste of our time.

So, this brings us to the decision making process—how do you make sound, solid decisions? We're faced with the need to make decisions every day—throughout the day. And we've all made some bad decisions, we sometimes wrestle with our decisions and sometimes change them back and forth. Have you ever had to make a decision, and you didn't know what to do and it stressed you out for days, weeks or months knowing that you needed to come to a conclusion? That's NO fun, is it? And how much time did you use during this process? Don't answer that. ☺

Making a decision gives us a sense of accomplishment—and remember, God gives us the right to choose. Okay, but again, how do you make sound, solid decisions and be content with them? How do you live a simple life when you can't make up your mind and tend to overcomplicate things?

We need to treat our decisions like our promises. We need to be COMMITTED to the decisions that we make, just as we're committed to the promises that we make. We are committed to our promises, right?

Let's look at how we should treat our word. In the olden days, people could make a contract simply by stating that they were going to do or sell something (give their word) and then shake hands on it. That settled it—the contract was sealed and they did whatever they committed to doing. They would say, "My word is my bond." Nowadays, contracts have to signed in front of lawyers and witnesses, and people tend to break (or try to break) contracts and then have to get additional lawyers to go to court and stand before a judge—just to keep their word! That shouldn't be.

If there's anything that I know—I KNOW THAT GOD IS FAITHFUL AND JUST TO PERFORM HIS WORD!!! I know it like I know my name! And He wants us to be people of our word as well. When you make a decision, it should be based on whether or not you can commit to the decision, and whether or not you can back it up with you actions. You're giving your word that you're going to do something.

Look at how God views His word:

In Isaiah 55:10-11, He says, "For as the rain comes down,
and the snow from heaven,
And does not return there,
But waters the earth,
And make it bring forth and bud,
That it may give seed to the sower
And bread to the eater,
11 So shall My word be that goes forth from My mouth;
It shall not return to Me void,
But it shall accomplish what I please,
And it shall prosper *in the thing* for which I sent it."

God is saying, whatever He says He's going to do—consider it done—He's not going to change His mind (or, in essence, change His word or decision.)

To live a simple life, you just need to be able to make sound decisions, and that should be based on what you can commit to and back up. You may be like me, an introvert, and need some time to process your thoughts in your mind before coming to a conclusion—that's okay, but when you come up with your decision, stick with it and see it through. You'll have accomplished one thing and will be ready for the next, thus able to get more done! Period.

Simple, isn't it?!

"Go confidently in the direction of your dreams! Live the life you've imagined. As you simplify your life, the laws of the universe will be simpler." Henry David Thoreau, 1817-1862, Author & Philosopher

Aleysha Recommends

Think about a decision that you have to make, whether a small or big one. Then think about the outcome or the end result based on whatever you decide.

Here's an example: you're undecided about buying a particular dress. Your decision about whether or not to make the purchase should be based on your COMMITMENT TO WEAR THE DRESS. Are you going to wear the dress after you buy it? If not, then leave it in the store.

Let's take for example the decision as to what new car you should purchase. Buy whatever car you can BE FAITHFUL TO MAKE THE MONTHLY PAYMENT ON.

It's really that simple.

In What Areas Would You Like to Improve?

Your Best Accessory

Hebrews 10:35: "Therefore, do not cast away your **confidence** which has great reward."

A person's best accessory is their confidence.

People are attracted to people with confidence. Not arrogance, but confidence. Why, you may ask? Because people like to connect themselves with others who are doing great things and going places in life. (Arrogance can have the opposite effect, and you may find people avoiding you like the plague.)

Confidence has a 'can do' attitude. And those whose confidence isn't at that level yet, will want to be connected to you to help build up their own confidence. They'll want to watch you and hear what you're saying so that they can duplicate it.

A truly confident person knows where their help comes from, and I'll give you a hint, it doesn't come from your own abilities, strength, education, bank account, college degrees or the like. Psalms 121: 1 says, "I will lift up my eyes to the hills—from where does my help come from? Verse 2: My help comes from the Lord, Who made heaven and earth."

People with confidence are positive, optimistic folks. No one likes being around someone who complains all of the time. Nor, someone who's shortsighted enough to think that their strength comes from themselves or another human being.

Confidence is an assurance that God is able at all times!

2 Corinthians 9:8 says, "And **God is able** to make **all** grace abound toward you, that you, always having **all** sufficiency in **all** things may have an abundance for **every** good work."

Take confidence in that—and in His Word!

Aleysha Recommends

What do you take confidence in? Is it a "power suit" while at the office—do you feel more confident when you're wearing your best suit? Do you take confidence in another person?

Think about how to "copy" those confident feelings in whatever you're wearing and no matter who's around you.

Also, pick up the pace in your walk. Confident people are busy people, and busy people tend to walk fast because they have places to go, people to see and things to do.

And learn to make eye contact with people. I once coached a business partner on being cognizant on making eye contact with people that she'd speak with. When she'd speak to them, she'd tend to not look them in the eye—her confidence level seemed to be so low. She confided in me that she wasn't very confident and didn't want people to stare her in the face. I shared with her that it was apparent that she wasn't confidence and needed to look people in the face to boost her confidence and thus, shorten the period of time she needed to speak with them.

Confidence says, "Okay, let me lay it out for you because I've got others who I need to share this information with too!"

Take confidence in knowing that God is ABLE to handle whatever concerns you today!

Wear your confidence well—it's your best accessory.

In What Areas Would You Like to Improve?

Strength While You're Waiting

The Prophet Isaiah knew something about waiting on the Lord. In Isaiah 40:30-31, he said, "Even the youth shall faint and be weary, and the young men shall utterly fall. Verse 31: But those who WAIT on the LORD. He shall renew their strength; they shall mount up with wings like eagles, they shall run and not be weary, they shall walk and not faint."

You'll find strength WHILE YOU'RE WAITING on the Lord! In today's modern super-quick, have to have it like yesterday world, there are some things that you're going to have to wait for. But the Lord promises that while you're waiting OH HIM, that He's going to RENEW YOUR STRENGTH!

Let's talk for a minute about eagles mounting up as verse 31 tells us. Eagles are about 3 feet long from head to foot—however their wingspan can reach up to 8 feet from wingtip to wingtip! Now, when an eagle mounts up—they aren't just doing it for nothing—THEY'RE GOING SOMEWHERE! They stretch out their long, magnificent wings and fly into the sky, ABOVE THE STORMS, and across the seas—again, they're going somewhere!

That's wonderful news! I'm so glad to know that while I'm waiting, while it may seem like it's taking a long time, I'm being strengthened during this time frame. It's during this time that you'll develop PATIENCE.

James 1:3 tells us, "Knowing that the testing of your faith produces patience. Verse 4: But let patience have its perfect work, that you may be perfect and complete, lacking nothing."

Do you want to be at peace and at ease? Then it's best to learn to have patience, it's a virtue! With patience, you don't pull your hair out when things are taking longer than you think that they should.

Do you want to mature in the things of God and be complete, lacking NOTHING? Then develop your patience. Knowing that while you're waiting and developing your patience, that the Lord is strengthening you!

Find something of worth to do while you're waiting. It's during these "time delays" that we can further develop our character, we can think on good or beautiful thoughts, we can learn to become optimistic and positive, we can work on our shortcomings, and we can draw closer to the Lord.

What have you got to lose?

It was while I was waiting on a specific prayer to be answered, which took about three months, that I wrote this book, built a new website, travelled out of town a few times to leadership retreats, spend time with family and friends, wrote a training program, got some rest and just enjoyed life. That's being quite productive during the time delays, wouldn't you say?

Consider a woman who's pregnant—it's during those nine months that she's PREPARING for the child that she's carrying. It's during that time that she sets up the nursery, buys clothes and toys for her forthcoming newborn, seeks out daycare providers, gets additional medical attention—she's quite busy while she's waiting. And look how mom and dad are being strengthened. Have you ever known a woman and/or a man who's a little afraid when they first find out that she's expecting? I have. But, a transformation takes place in that nine month waiting period—they're being strengthened to be loving and careful parents of this new life that's being brought into the world. Their confidence level goes up several notches.

Are you "pregnant" with a dream, "pregnant" with a prayer that's been in your heart? Make sure you prepare for the answer while you're waiting for it to manifest in your life.

Ecclesiastes 5:3 says, "For a dream comes through much activity, and a fool's voice is known by his many words."

Be busy while you're waiting.

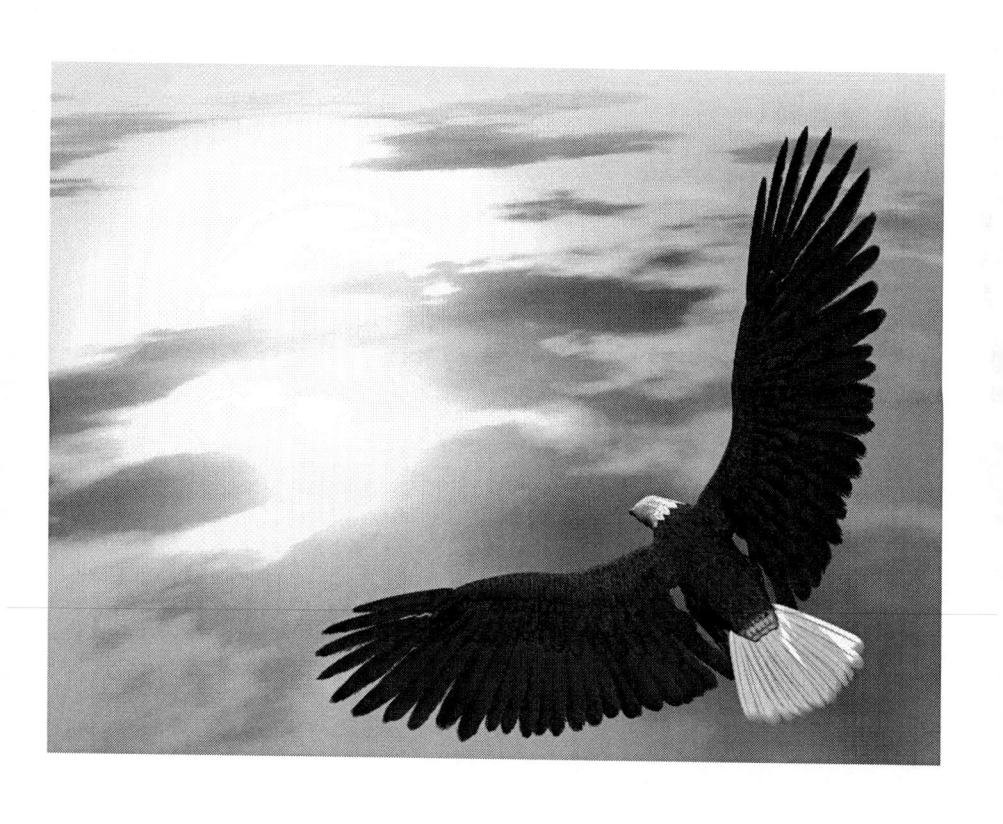

Aleysha Recommends

What prayers are you waiting to be answered? What can you do in the meantime to prepare for the answer? Be busy while you're waiting.

Keep in mind, you're preparing yourself for the answer to your prayers during the waiting period, not trying to rush it along.

In What Areas Would You Like to Improve?

Oh—To Be Thankful!

Is anyone grateful today?!

1 Chronicles 16:34 says, "Oh, give **thanks** to the Lord, for He is good! For His mercy endures forever."

Gratitude will take you far in life! We've all heard that your attitude will determine your altitude. Let me also say that your GRATITUDE will determine your altitude!

Giving thanks is mentioned over 100 times in the Bible.

The Bible says that we are to come before the Lord with THANKSGIVING! God doesn't like complaining and grumbling, but He loves it when you give Thanks—give thanks in everything!

Do you remember the ten men who had the awful disease of leprosy who came to Jesus and He healed all of them?

Luke 17:11 says, "Now it happened as He went to Jerusalem that He passed through the midst of Samaria and Galilee. **12** Then as He entered a certain village, there met Him ten men who were lepers, who stood afar off. **13** And they lifted up *their* voices and said, "Jesus, Master, have mercy on us!" **14** So when He saw *them,* He said to them, "Go, show yourselves to the priests." And so it was that **as they went, they were cleansed. 15 And one of them,** when he saw that he was healed, returned, and with a loud voice glorified God, **16** and fell down on *his* face at His feet, giving Him thanks. And he was a Samaritan. **17** So Jesus answered and said, **"Were there not ten cleansed? But where *are* the other nine? 18** Were there not any found who returned to give glory to God except this foreigner?" **19** And He said to the one man, "Arise, go your way. Your faith has made you well."

Gratitude is so important to the Lord that He said in Verse 17, "Weren't there ten men who were cleansed, so then where are the other nine to say thank you?"

Of course the Lord knows the thoughts and feelings that we have. He knew that the other nine men who were healed of such a horrible disease HAD to be thankful that they were now cleansed, but He wanted to hear it. And today, He still wants to hear our gratitude. Look at what He said about the one man who came back to give thanks, "Arise, go your way. Your faith has made you well."

Are you suffering from an illness or condition today? Give the Lord thanks for the healing that He's already provided! Are you suffering from a lack of resources? Give the Lord thanks for what He's already provided!

Gratitude will make room for more blessings to come into your life. Have you ever given something to someone and they were just so genuinely thankful that you wanted to give them even more? Why? Because their level of gratitude had a major impact on your heart!

Remember, gratitude will determine your altitude!

A friend once shared this email with me, after I tweaked it a little bit, I was just blown away with it!

"From a strictly Mathematical Viewpoint:

What Equals 100%? What does it mean to give MORE than 100%? Ever wonder about those people who say they are giving more than 100%? We have all been in situations where someone wants you to give over 100%. How about achieving 101%? What equals 100% in life?

Here's a little mathematical formula that might help you answer these questions:

If:
A B C D E F G H I J K L M N O P Q R S T U V W X Y Z

Is represented as:
1 2 3 4 5 6 7 8 9 10 11 12 13 14 15 16 17 18 1 9 20 21 22 23 24 25 26.

Then:

K-N-O-W-L-E-D-G-E
11+14+15+23+12+5+4+7+5 = 96%

We're getting close to that 100% goal!

And:

H-A-R-D-W-O-R-K
8+1+18+4+23+15+18+11 = 98%

We're getting closer!

But,

A-T-T-I-T-U-D-E
1+20+20+9+20+21+4+5 = 100%

Ah ha! We're there!

But for those who want to go beyond giving 100%, remember, we talked about the EXTRA-ORDINARY!

Let's look at this:

G-R-A-T-I-T-U-D-E
7+18+1+20+9+20+21+4+5=105%!!!

Therefore, one can conclude with mathematical certainty that: While Knowledge and Hard Work will get you close, and Attitude will get you there, it's Gratitude that will put you over the top!" Isn't that interesting?!

Aleysha Recommends

As the old hymn says, "Count your blessings, name them one by one. Count your blessings, see what God has done!"

Take stock of everything that you have to be grateful for—and give thanks for things that will get better, as if it already has!

Gratitude makes room for new blessings to come into your life.

In What Areas Would You Like to Improve?

The Wellness Factor

1 Corinthians 6:18-20 says, "Do you not know that your body is the temple of the Holy Spirit *who is* in you, whom you have from God, and you are not your own? 20 For you were bought at a price; therefore glorify God in your body and in your spirit, which are God's."

The Lord is very particular about you! You're His temple!! King David said in Psalms 139:14, that we are fearfully and wonderfully made—MARVELOUS are His works! God is so particular about you that there's NO ONE who looks exactly like you, NO ONE has your same DNA or fingerprints, NO ONE has your same likes and dislikes. Do you remember in the Old Testament of the Bible when they would build a temple to the Lord—not just anyone could build a temple, God Himself selected those who would do so.

King David, Solomon's father, deeply wanted to build a temple for the Lord, but God said to David in I Chronicles 22:8, "You have shed much blood and have made great wars; you shall not build a house for My name, because you have shed much blood on the earth in My sight. Verse 9: Behold a son shall be born to you, who shall be a man of REST; and I will give him rest from all of his enemies all around. His name shall be Solomon. Verse 10: He shall build a house for My name."

King David, although he couldn't build the Lord's temple, did make very valuable donations to it. He said that the temple for the Lord must be EXCEEDINGLY MAGNIFICENT, FAMOUS AND GLORIOUS throughout all countries, and he would make preparation for it. (I Chronicles 22:5b).

Now, check out what King David donated to the Lord's exceedingly magnificent, famous and glorious temple:

I Chronicles 29:2 "Now for the house of my God I have prepared with all my might: gold for *things to be made of* gold, silver for *things of* silver, bronze for *things of* bronze, iron for *things of* iron, wood *for things of* wood, onyx stones, *stones* to be set, glistening stones of various colors, all kinds of precious stones, and marble slabs in abundance. Verse 3 Moreover, because I have set my affection on the house of my God, I have given to the house of my God, over and above all that I have prepared for the holy house, my own special treasure of gold and silver: Verse 4 three thousand talents of gold, of the gold of Ophir, and seven thousand talents of refined silver, to overlay the walls of the houses; Verse 5 the gold for *things of* gold and the silver for *things of* silver, and for all kinds of work *to be done* by the hands of craftsmen. Who *then* is willing to consecrate himself this day to the LORD?"

You see, the Lord's temple was not a piece of junk, and neither are you (modern day temple of the Lord!) Anyone who has accepted Christ into their lives, is now a walking temple for the Lord.

And with that said, we have to do some temple maintenance and upkeep!

If you're not going to take care of your own body, then who is? You've heard the saying, "Your health is your wealth!" We don't bring glory to God in run-down, sick bodies. Many sicknesses that people suffer can be prevented.

Let's talk about your physical temple for a minute. I would like for you to consider the wellness factor and have routine medical check-ups done. Including, pap smears, mammograms, physicals, prostate checks (for men), dental exams and eye exams.

Also, rest your temple. God said that Solomon would be a man of rest—and we talked about resting in our "How to Be" chapter.

Let me also encourage you to drink at least 8 glasses of water each day. Our bodies mainly consist of water and crave to be hydrated. Don't be a disservice to your physical temple by keeping it dehydrated—go ahead and have some water to drink. You'll be so glad that you did—it has lots of benefits such as clear skin, a flushed out system, helps in weight loss and more.

Go ahead, and keep the Lord's temple EXCEEDINGLY MAGNIFICENT, FAMOUS AND GLORIOUS!

Aleysha Recommends

You have to take great care of yourself (your temple, God's temple!)

- Schedule your annual or routine pap smears, mammograms, dental cleanings and check-ups, physicals, eye exams, etc.

- Drink at least 8 glasses of water per day.

- Get 6-8 hours of sleep per night.

- Take a daily supplement or multivitamin.

- Exercise—even if it's just walking a few extra steps per day by taking the stairs instead of the elevator—do something.

- Be good to yourself!

In What Areas Would You Like to Improve?

. . . and Amen

1 Peter 5:10-11 says, "May the God of all *grace,* Who called us to His eternal glory by Christ Jesus, after you have suffered (waited) a while, may He perfect, establish, strengthen, and settle you. To Him be the glory and the dominion forever and ever. Amen."

Have you ever met someone who was attractive on the outside, only to get to know them and their beauty and good looks start to wane? Or maybe you've met someone who you didn't think was good looking and spent some time with that person and they turned out to be beautiful? I'm sure that you have—on many occasions. Therefore, we can determine that beauty, style and grace are really determined by what's going on inside of us—not solely the outward appearance.

Now, you have an idea of what your personal style is and what colors are best for you. However, before we can dress the outside and make it look beautiful, we REALLY have to work on our insides. Beauty, style and grace really DOES start on the inside and then it shows up on the outside.

Don't try to dress a mess. Fix the "real" you up first, and the outer fixing up becomes easy!

It's my prayer that this book will help you to live a more balanced life.

And be encouraged—THERE'S HOPE!

God Bless You!

So, let's summarize what we've talked about:

What is Style? It's being yourself on purpose.

What is Grace? It's provision, it's favor, it's a gift from God!

How to BE (and rest!)

What Are You Thinking About? You are what you're consistently thinking about!

The Spirit of Excellence—Everyone can have it, it's just a matter of choice!

The Beauty of Creating—God has given you the ability to create the life that you want!

A Leader Worth Following—It starts with a servant's heart—and leading is made possible with an understanding heart.

The Simple Life—Simplify your life by making good decisions.

Your Best Accessory—Is your confidence!

Strength While You're Waiting—Bask in the fact that you're being prepared! There's hope during the time delays.

Oh—To Be Thankful! God is looking for someone who's thankful and continues to bless those who bless Him with gratitude!

The Wellness Factor—Your health is your wealth!

. . . and AMEN—Amen!

Aleysha R. Proctor

Aleysha Proctor is a professional, certified Image Consultant. She studied with Color Me Beautiful, Beauty for All Seasons and Brenda York's Image Management. She also has a BS degree in Management and Leadership from Kennedy Western University and an MBA in Marketing from Hamilton University.

Aleysha is an Independent Consultant with Warm Spirit, Inc., the self-care & wellness company. She won the company's 2006 Top Living to Your Potential award and the 2006 Cornerstone of Success award. She also leads a very productive team in the company's #1 state for sales (Maryland).

She's been quoted in publications such as *Black Enterprise, Prince George's County Suite, Washingtonian, Empowering Women* and *Onyx Woman* magazines on topics such as image, beauty, business & lifestyle.

She has a career working with the nation's power brokers on Capitol Hill in Washington, DC.

Aleysha is a member of ISES (International Special Events Society), FGI (Fashion Group International) and First Baptist Church of Glenarden Maryland.

Her passion in life is helping others to live their best lives now by realizing and utilizing their gifts and potential!

For more information, visit
www.AleyshaProctor.com.